How to Stop Yo-Yo Dieting

Avoid the Ups and Downs

By Elaina Moore

Table of Contents:

It's Not Your Fault...the Dieting Industry has Set You Up to Fail

It consumes you. It's there every single minute of every single day. It's that nagging knowing inside that you need to lose weight. You need to get in shape. You should be on a diet right now. Well...you are on one, it's just the candy bar in one hand and the Coca-Cola in the other that's the problem. You've blown it...again!

But what the heck, right? "I'll start a new diet tomorrow", you tell yourself. And since you've made such a mess of this diet, might as well have a donut to go with the candy bar. I mean...what difference does it make anyway? You're feel like a loser.

Does this sound familiar? Do you constantly struggle with your weight? You eat a piece of cake and you swear you can see it on your thighs already. The sweeter the chocolate, the worse the remorse. The guilt sets in and then the hopelessness. What does it matter now? And the circle goes on, and on...and on and the stress just adds on more pounds.

Does the mere mention of starting yet another "diet" stress you out? But you desperately want to be lean, sexy, healthy, vibrant and full of life?

Let me put your mind at ease. Diets don't work. They make you fat and keep you fat. "Dieting" is a state of mind that demands failure and stirs up feelings of guilt and hopelessness. And worse yet…the "diet gurus" that come out with a new infomercial, new book, new miracle pill, etc… seemingly every week are lying to you! Yes, I said that….they are lying to you! They push all your hot buttons to get you buy their next program so they keep up their income with little regard to the results you will actually achieve.

It's time to find a new way to a new you… without all the ups and downs of "dieting"! I'm going to show you how to break though that mentally and physically inside of this book. When's the last time you stood in front of a full length mirror and liked what you saw? That's what I want for you! That's what you can achieve by reading and applying the principles in this book.

I believe you! Let's do this together!

Elaina Moore

By the way, I want to reach as many people as possible with this message of "How to Stop Yo-Yo Dieting so please don't forget to leave this book a 5 start review on Amazon!

STRAIGHT TALK ABOUT WEIGHT LOSS AND DIETING

Does dieting make you fat? It sure seems like it sometimes. At the best, starting a diet is just setting yourself up to fail. Right? And what do most of us do when we fail? Exactly!

But it doesn't have to be that way. Knowledge is power and what you're going to learn in this book will knock your socks off…and some pounds too. Read on to find out all you need to know about what doesn't work and to discover what does!

Give yourself a break. There's a good reason why you fall face first into an apple pie every time you "diet". It has been scientifically proven that diets do not work. In fact, they do worse. They make you fat. Not all dieters find that to be true but the majority rule is that most diets lead to weight gain.

When is the last time you put your sock on inside out? You probably have no idea and it most likely makes no difference to you. You have learned that if you put socks on inside out, you just turn them to the right side and put them on again. Simple as that. There is no need to obsess on possibly putting them on wrong again, endlessly fixated on others who seem to have their socks on correctly. It's just not a big deal.

I have a friend who used to have a problem with alcohol. It almost ruined her life. She is clean and sober now so I recently asked her how long it had been since she took a drink. "I'm not sure," she answered, honestly. "Let me count. Six years!" She went on to tell me that drinking is no longer something she thinks about. It is just part of her life anymore. Six years had come and gone but yet she was not counting the days. That is when knew that she was truly free.

When is the last time you had a big thick luscious bite of cherry pie dripping with melted vanilla ice cream? When was the last time you even took a nibble of a chocolate bar or a sinful taste of a donut? Chances are that you can tell me the day and probably even the time that you indulged. Why? Because you are consumed with not doing it. How's that working for you?

The object of this book is not to give free reign to poor eating habits. Poor eating habits will make you fat and can lead to serious illnesses. Neither is the aim to get you to quit exercising or to not do anything to control the way that your body looks. It is, in fact, quite the opposite. The goal of what you are about to discover is to teach you a new way of thinking, a new way of living so that you can be free.

The reasons why diets are a "set up" are both physical and physiological. In this book you will find out why and also, that it is not your fault. You no longer have to feel guilty and drown those feelings in yet another chocolate cake. You don't have to feel deprived and give in to that big bowl of ice cream to even the score. So, take the pressure of dieting off yourself and learn the secrets of becoming a new you, from the inside out.

Before we go any further, you really need to take to heart that you are beautiful the way you are. The pounds we put on usually tell a story, the pages of our lives. Did you put on some pounds in college while eating junk food and nervously snacking while cramming for exams? Maybe the baby fat you took on during pregnancy just never went away. Life happens and it's not all bad. It's fantastic and very healthy to want to lose weight and get in shape but in order to do so, it's imperative to love and accept yourself, just the way you are.

Body Typing (Getting Comfortable with "You")

Knowing your body type is key to figuring out what your target weight and shape should be. Its also the first step in eliminating yo-yo dieting. Wondering what types have to do with yo-yo dieting? Let me explain....If you're a endomorph but trying to look like your favorite ectomorph movie start, your efforts are in vain. No matter how much you diet like her, work out like her and try to be like here, you get her results because you have different body types. You see every body type has specific type of eating, specific type of workout, specific lifestyle plan to help them optimize their figure. Where most people set themselves up for a huge failure following a diet and workout plan based around someone else's body type. Then when it doesn't work or they don't look the person they are trying to model after you become disappointed, quit and then move on to trying the next "diet". Make sense? Okay great…so it's about optimizing your body for your personal body type.

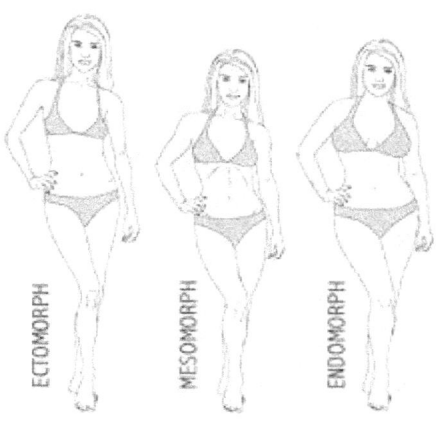

Now before we get into the body types its important to know there are positive things about each of the body types and negative things as well. No one type is perfect. Keep in mind that the goal here is to improve on what you have and to work with what you've got.

Basically, everyone falls into one of three body types: Ectomorph, Mesomorph, or Endomorph. Some have a combination of two, one on their upper body and another on their lower or some variance. You should be able to spot the one or ones that best describe your body pretty easily.

An Ectomorph body type is usually skinny by nature. If you are an Ectomorph, you might have been made fun of in school. "If you turn sideways and stick out your tongue, you'd look like a zipper," kids might have teased. But it's alright. Those same kids grew up to be adults that are now very envious. This body type usually has a great metabolism and finds it difficult to gain weight. Their chest, shoulders and derriere are generally small and typically they are energetic and sometimes even hyper.

Ectomorphs

Bodily Characteristics

- Smaller bone structure
- Thin limbs
- Small shoulders, chest and buttocks
- Difficulty building muscle
- High metabolism
- High Carbohydrate Tolerance

Ectomorphs make great endurance racers. Due to their low fat and lean muscle distribution coupled with their endless energy, they are generally the ones you see wining a marathon or jumping hurdles with little effort. They play a mean game of basketball and can run a ball down the soccer field in no time flat. Because they have a hard time building muscle, they aren't usually found in the gym doing bodybuilding, but the muscle they do have works well for them when it comes to speed.
As far as personality typing, Ectomorphs are thought to be fearful and timid though often hyperactive as children. They are also said to be intellectual. Of course, those things do not always hold true but is a typical stereo-typing of an Ectomorph.

Ectomorph women are no exception. They are often marathon runners, endurance racers and roller derby queens. They may end up being high fashion models because of their slender build.

If that one doesn't sound familiar, we'll keep on moving. The Mesomorph is an athletic build. This one is also called the "hourglass figure". Naturally lean and muscly the Mesomorph generally has medium sized joints and a descent metabolism. They gain weight but it is evenly distributed. Losing weight comes easy for a Mesomorph and gaining muscle comes with little effort as well.

Mesomorphs

- Medium bone structure
- Muscle bound limbs
- Broad shoulders
- High muscle throughout body
- Build muscle easily
- Burn fat easily
-

Mesomorphs tend to be average framed individuals with lots of muscles. They are able to build muscle fairly easily and have little trouble losing fat because they burn fat with their strong muscles. Mesomorphs are likely to be football players, bodybuilders, strong swimmers, wrestlers and boxers. Females often excel in gymnastics, cheerleading and female boxing if they have a good mind to do so.

Mesomorphs are often stereo-typed as popular individuals that excel in sports and anything else they determine to do. They are thought to be strong-willed and bull-headed. One thing is for sure, you do not want to push the buttons of a Mesomorph.

It is when a Mesomorph stops being active that trouble can set in. If they are not burning fat with their muscles, it accumulates. Heart disease are cardiovascular issues can plague an inactive Mesomorph.

Still not you? The Endomorph body type is curvier and is sometimes referred to as a "Pear Shape" because of their small shoulders cast against a high waistline and over-sized hips can resemble that of a pear. Gaining weight comes easily for the Endomorph but taking it off, not so much.

Endomorphs

- **Large Bone Structure**
- **Tendency to Retain Fat**
- **Difficulty in Losing Weight**
- **Gain Weight Easily**

Endomorphs are those huge guys you see on TV, lifting unbelievable amounts of weight and doing incredible feats with their bare strength coupled with their size. That is if you can get them to do it. An Endomorph is sometimes considered to be lazy and sloppy, perhaps unmotivated. Once they set their mind to do something, though, they generally have the capability to.

You do not want to come across an Endomorph on the football field if you are on the opposing team. He is the lineman to watch out for. Endomorphs make great sumo wrestlers. A female Endomorph might be a female wrestler or the goalie in soccer.

Endomorphs have a tough go of dieting. Stereo-typed as being sluggish, that is not always the case and certainly not the general rule as far as weight loss. They simply have a harder time ridding their body of fat and accumulating muscle that burns the fat. It is easy for an Endomorph to be discouraged, especially if he or she is comparing themselves with another body type.

Nature plays a big part in predetermining how our body is proportioned. Hormones do too. Those who tend to gain in the buttocks and hips and have saddlebags are a product of the evolution of a woman's body due to fertility and breast feeding.

Once you have identified your shape, you can set reachable goals in mind. You can focus on areas that your body type tends to have trouble with but you can also give yourself a break, knowing that if you are an Endomorph, you will never be an Ectomorph and visa-versa. After all, a banana would look funny shaped like an apple, wouldn't it? The same is true with humans and our body types.

Understanding your body type or types and how you personally respond to different foods and different workouts.

So keep reading because we'll dive into how to optimize your nutrition and workouts for your body type later in the book.

Waist-To-Hip Calculation

Instead of hitting the scales, a better way to determine how much weight, or fat, you should lose can be calculated by body fat percentage or the the waist-to-hip ratio method. Since you probably don't have a spare set of body fat calipers laying around we going to use the waist to hip ratio.

Here's how to take your measurements. Simply measure your waist, right at your belly button. Then measure the widest part of your hips. Divide the measurement of your waist by the measurement of your hips and you have your waist-to-hip ratio. Medical institutions have set 0.80 for women and 0.95 for men as the best ratio but again, go at it realistically.

One thing is for sure and for certain, if you follow the steps outlined in this book you will begin to see results. This book will help you piece it all together and get your inner-self on the right track so that you can do exactly that.

The more you know about yourself and your personal body type or types, the more realistic it will be to stop the madness of dieting only to gain weight and flood yourself with guilt and the easier it will be to make great strides. Remember its progress, not perfection that holds the key.

There is no magic formula so for heaven's sake, put down those green coffee beans and acai pills that cost a small fortune and never work anyway. Set your mind realistically, embrace who you are and THEN you can get excited about the shape of things to come.

THE "ROOT" OF YOUR WEIGHT LOSS AND DIETING PROBLEM

Before you can expect a real change what lies on the outside, you have to take a look at what lies within. On the hit television reality series, "The Biggest Loser", you might note that as the layers of flab begin to fall, it is almost inevitable that the person behind the pounds becomes extremely vulnerable emotionally. Things buried way inside have been covered and are being exposed. It is often uncomfortable for the person as it may be for you as well but it's time to take a good look at the inner you.

Did you know that eating disorders can date back to early childhood and perhaps even to the months spent in the womb? Prospective foster parents are schooled to watch for abnormal eating patterns such as a youngster who will consume anything and everything put before him or her and still scrounge for more. They are also advised to watch for food hoarding. Although the child's stomach is completely full, the need for the comfort it brings cannot be quenched.

"Comfort food" is a phrase coined to describe some foods that are especially satisfying because they are homemade or made in large quantities or even because they are of a certain ethnic group, like Italian. But the truth is that for some, food in general is comforting. Children who have gone hungry tend to find comfort in food but others do as well. Sometimes food is a padding for other emotional issues such as not feeling loved, being jealous or fearful thoughts.

Lack of control is another obvious reason for overeating. While it is easy to think it is just a weakness, there are other philosophies that approach it differently. William Herbert taught that an Endomorphic body and personality type would be prone to indulge in food.

Others attest that another reason for eating disorders is the feeling of being in control. It is common for teen-age girls, and older ones as well, to judge their identity on their personal appearance and often go overboard on trying to regulate their food intake, resulting in such conditions as Anorexia Nervosa, Bulimia Nervosa and Binging.

It is also thought that some even purposefully overeat to make a statement. A young girl who is being sexually abused may think that being overweight will stop the abuse. Some women have even admitted to getting fat as a child to be like a parent or sibling who was obese.

No matter what the reason behind it is, overeating is often emotionally stemmed. You may know that you have an issue behind your weight gain, or you may suspect that you do. Weight loss and getting in shape comes from the inside out. It begins in your mind and in your emotions as well. It is of upmost importance to examine the very depths of the inner you to determine if there is a link and if there is…there is help.

Stress

Did you know that stress can make you fat? It sure can. Knowing that is enough to stress anyone out. It is all caused by a chemical reaction that takes place when your body senses danger. It's the old "fight or flight" syndrome. When in a situation your body considers dangerous, a stress hormone call cortisol shoots out causing a rush of adrenalin and other changes in the body designed to make you faster so you can deal with the danger at hand.

The problem is that in our world today, much of our stress is not the kind that requires us to run through the jungle or fight a bear with our bare hand. With no place to go, the cortisol sits around in the body and can cause "chronic stress" leading to an imbalance of blood sugar, metabolism issues and even increased hunger.

Certain areas in our bodies tend to hold in fat caused by stress such as the belly and around the hips. Instead of stressing on being stressed, it's a good idea to find out what your stress triggers are and to do all you can to deal with them constructively.

How to Avoid all the "Emotional Traps" (The ones that cause additional eating and Weight Gain)

Identify Your Emotional Triggers:

We all do it, to some extent. We set ourselves up to fail, especially when it comes to a diet or exercise plan. We set outrageous goals and then beat ourselves up when we don't reach them.

There are other destructive patterns we may fall into as well. Do you do great with your diet for a week or two, maybe even a month, only to go on a binge that undoes everything? Or maybe you eat when you are bored, or depressed or when you are angry. You get the picture. Identifying what exactly makes you "fall off the wagon" and discovering why you do what you do is priceless. Finding the problem is the first step to finding the solution.

So next step is try and identify what emotional triggers are that are causing you to overeat, to quit a diet, to become stressed out, to feel out of control,etc...

Go ahead and think about that now. Right them down.

Now that you recognize what goes on in your head before you self sabotage your dieting efforts you can be aware of it next time it happens and push through it. In some cases you may not be able to push though it on your own by just recognizing it's there so here are some great ways to address all the "emotional traps" you might find yourself in.

AVOIDING THE UPS AND DOWNS

Motivation

Getting to the weight you want to be at is going to take effort. Most good things in life do. That is why simply taking a pill or eating a grapefruit just don't work. In order to get up off the couch and do something about the shape you are in, you'll need some motivation.

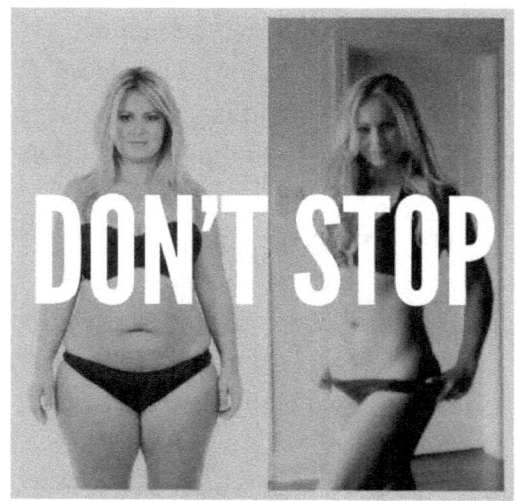

Motivation is what kicks you into gear. What gets you going? Does seeing a poster of a perfect 10 model give you the gumption to improve yourself? For a lot of us, hearing a story about someone a lot like us who overcame and lost weight is more encouraging.

Maybe for you, a picture of your child or significant other makes you want to see results. Or, maybe music sets you in motion. Whatever it is that inspires you and gets those positive thoughts rolling that fuel your fire, do it! Results require action and action requires motivation.

Personally I like to keep a picture of someone who is my "ideal" physique on my bathroom mirror so that I'm reminded every day to stay motivated. Sometimes before/after pictures of someone you think made great body transformation is good motivation. It's a reminder that it does take work to have an awesome body and that other people do work for it! Even those movie stars that always look great work for the body they have!

So find your motivation and keep it in front of you!

If something big, bad and ugly was after you, chances are you'd stop at nothing to get away from it. You'd leap tall buildings in a single bound or run through fire. The same is true for things we really want. We usually find a way to get what we really truly want. Purpose in your heart just how bad you want results and picture it done. Embrace that picture and hold it to heart. Tear down the walls that come between you now and the new you that you wish to see.

Commitment

Some people are downright afraid to commit to anything. I have heard a number of people say that if they dare mention that they are dieting, it is sure to backfire. While that may be true in a self-destructive course, commitment can be seen as a good thing too.

Just think, if you were not committed to paying your bills, you might not get around to it and there you'd be without power, a phone and maybe even a place to live. Commitment keeps us bound to an agreement and a life-style change, such as a diet plan, certainly could use some grounding when the going gets tough because, it will.

It is up to you if you mention your plan to anyone, but do make a personal commitment and hold yourself to it. Write it down. Stick it on the fridge. Start a blog or a diary. Do whatever you need to do to stick with it.

Rewards

Human nature is based on the reward system. We do what works. When kids throw a temper tantrum, they do it because…it works. We work to get a paycheck. We are even nice to people because it makes us feel good. There is always a pay-off. It's a fact but it's not necessarily a bad thing, it's just human nature. Keeping that in mind, be sure to reward yourself for a job well done. If you reach a goal, go enjoy a movie with a friend or even treat yourself to a manicure or if it's a real milestone, check in for a day at the spa. While it is alright to give yourself permission to cheat once a week, once a month or whatever works for you, it is best to not use food as a reward.

The Fall

You're going to fall sometimes. It's just a fact. You are human and unless you know a secret that no one else does, chances are good that you are going to fail at one point or another. Remember though that failure is never final. Dust off and move forward. It's not how many times you fall that count, it's how many times you get back up. Many of life's most important lessons are learned from what might be otherwise be considered failures. Remember Thomas Edison failed 1000 times when attempting to invent the light bulb. But in his mind, he found 1000 ways that didn't work. It's all about how you look at things that will take you where you want to go. Attitude is everything and getting right back up is…imperative.

Finding Help

For many of you, the information and inspiration found in this book will be enough to motivate you to achieve great results. Others, however, may need a little more help. If you think that you may have an issue with eating, there is nothing shameful about seeking help. In fact, it is quite the contrary. It is taking charge so that you can change the shape that your body, and your life, are in.

Books

Tons of fantastic books have been written on the psychology of overeating. While this books touches on various aspects, there are entire books devoted to specific issues. Eating disorders, sex abuse issues, and a myriad of other topics are available online and in hard copy. It is well worth checking out what experts in the field have to offer.

Counselors

If you have deep-rooted issues that you feel are holding you back from going forward, by all means, see a professional. That is what they are there for. Sometimes it helps just to talk about it and vent. Together, you may work it out in just one or two visits. If it takes longer, that's alright too. You wouldn't deny help to your child, mate or best friend, would you? Don't deny it to yourself either. It's all party of loving and nurturing the inner you.

Groups

Some of us are just group people. We work better in a group whether it is exercising, dieting or talking about psychological issues with food. It makes us accountable, for one thing. It also helps us feel better to find we are not alone.

If you feel you have an eating addiction, there are support groups such as Overeaters Anonymous that offers a 12 step program which includes a sponsor who has "been there and done that" who can help walk you through it. As the name implies, it is totally confidential.

Alternative Methods

More and more, people are turning to non-traditional forms of help for issues such as overeating when will power is not enough. Many of the methods were very popular in ancient times and are making a huge come back these days. Only you can determine if you would like to give one a try. Keep in mind that these practices are to get you over a hurdle and not to cure you. They are designed to help you help yourself.

With deep roots in the ancient Orient, acupuncture offers much in the way of food addictions and other issues that may stand in the way of your diet and work-out program. Administered by sticking needles under the skin, the intent of acupuncture is to open up blocked energy (qi) passages so your body can function properly. It is also said that it gives you energy which is conducive when it comes to exercising.

Acupressure is another option. It works along the same lines, opening up clogged energy channels, but uses carefully articulated pressure from fingertips, elbows or another body part or device to do the job rather than using needles. Many find this procedure less invasive than being pricked with needles. You can even be taught to perform acupressure on yourself.

Ayurveda is an alternative medical practice widely used by the Indian culture for hundreds of years and presently as well. The goal with Ayurveda is to find a balance of the body, mind and spirit. The practice is becoming quite popular, especially in the weight loss area, due in part to the popular alternative doctor, Dr. John Douillard, who has been promoting Ayurveda for years.

A number of people with weight issues are turning to Chiropractic measures for help with their weight. Subluxations, according to Chiropractors, can lead to eating disorders and can even play a role in faulty weight distribution. There are two types of Chiropractors. One accommodates those who simply need an adjustment and the other focuses more on life issues such as weight loss solutions.

Hypnosis is certainly worth checking into if you are obsessed with food or with thoughts of food, good and bad. Hypnotherapy is basically coming to peace with your inner self to overcome a problem. It can be done with the help of a hypnotherapist or can be achieved on your own, often with the aid of an audio prop or even a book. It is gaining popularity for many who have issues with stress, drugs, alcohol, cigarettes and weight loss too.

IS MY WEIGHT GAIN REALLY A MEDICAL REASON? (HERE'S HOW TO FIND OUT)

Medical Issues

Medical issues can lead to gaining weight and gaining weight can lead to medical issues. It's an endless cycle. If you suspect you have an underlying medical problem that is either stemming from your weight gain or causing your weight gain, be sure to consult with your physician. Diabetes, thyroid issues and even cancer can contribute to weight problems.

If you do have a medical problem, it is not a deal breaker. You can adjust your eating and exercise plan to incorporate your doctor's recommendations. Many ailments actually motivate people to make changes that actual make them healthier. It's a matter of what you do with the information at hand that will determine the outcome.

Aside from common things like diabetes that you doctor might readily address many people suffer from thyroid or hormone imbalances that causing out of control weight gain.

Luckily there is an easy way to find out if either of these are an issue for you!

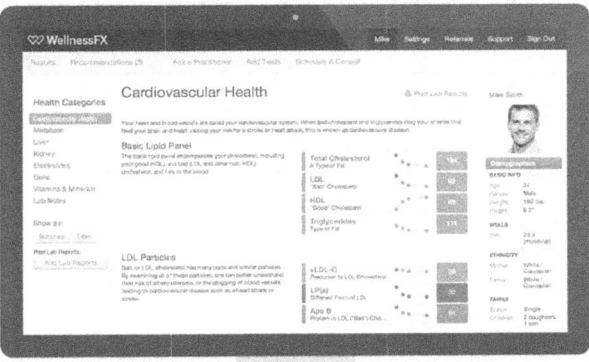 All you need to do is a thyroid and hormone panel though a company called

WellnessFX.com

It just requires a very easy and inexpensive blood test to find out if your real issue is with your thyroid or hormones. They have a very simple dashboard feature that shows you if your numbers are red(for bad), yellow(for okay) and green(good). They even have coaches to help you understand your blood work results and how to improve your numbers if they are off.

Milestones

There are times in our lives that we can be expected to put on a few pounds. Giving birth to a child, then perhaps a second or third and going through menopause are all occasions when most will add some weight. You may have to work harder to lose those pounds and sometimes it is just time to accept it. A mother of four will not have her sixteen year-old body back and a woman of sixty will never look eighteen. Neither are we supposed to. If your belly bulges because it has been stretched with twins or if your hips are widening because you have reached menopause, certainly give those trouble spots some extra TLC but don't obsess on them. Like body typing, we all must milestone type our bodies as well and as the old prayer goes we must have the serenity to accept that what we cannot change, the courage to change the things we can and the wisdom to know the difference.

EAT RIGHT FOR YOUR BODY TYPE

You may be asking yourself why you need to seek help or be motivated at all if there is no diet to follow. Think back to your socks. While putting them on inside out is not something that consumes your thoughts and causes a daily struggle, you still do it, probably each and every day. The same with my friend. She no longer counts the hours or days or even years since her last drink, she simply does not drink. But discovering how to free yourself and how to put healthy thoughts and actions into your life does take knowledge, motivation and action.

Once you are to that point, it is time to learn what does work. Keep in mind that what works for one, may not work for the other. Know your body type, your medical issues and psychological state. Search your soul. Finding the right weight management plan or combination of plans that is tailored for you is key. After all, it's all about you, right?

Food 101

Back in the day, weight was not the huge issue it is these days. People ate off the land, worked hard and stayed fit. For the most part. In many cultures in the olden days, it was desirable to be fat. It was a thing of clout, a statement. It meant that you were well enough to lay around and eat bon-bons.

Much has changed and being overweight is no longer a fashion statement. We all want to look fit and trim. But we can learn from the men and women of old, beginning with what they did and didn't eat.

Hunger

There's nothing worse than being hungry and not being able to eat. In fact, it's so cruel, it is a favored torture for prisoner camps. In my mother's Living Will, she clearly stated Do Not Resuscitate but included a clause that she was not to be starved under any circumstance. Being hungry is…not good.

The promise of eating correctly is that you don't have to be hungry. Your body has an automatic switch in it that tells you when to start eating and when to stop. But, you have to get healthy enough to tune in on it and, you must eat the right foods.

Protein

Protein has become the catch phrase in diet fads. You have your protein shakes and your protein bars, the protein diet plan and protein potion pills. So what's the big deal about protein?
Proteins are that important. They contain nutrients that our bodies must have to maintain and repair. They play a huge role in the health of your immune system and determine the well-being of your hormones too. Furthermore, proteins help to fill you up and make you actually feel full, unlike junk food that does the opposite.

One reason proteins are so vital is that they contain amino acids, twenty-two of them to be exact. Amino acids are vital to have in order to be healthy. Only fourteen of the twenty-two can be produced by the body. They remaining eight must come from what you eat. Complete, true protein is the only source in which we can find them. The key word is complete. Not all proteins are created alike. Meat eggs, cheese and foods that are made from animal derivatives constitute complete proteins. They are the only proteins that contribute the eight missing essential amino acids, in other words. Other proteins are important but do not leave out those that you must have in order to maintain your amino acid levels.

In order to feel full and be healthy, protein is a must. One grave mistake dieters make is cutting calories to the point that their body gleans protein from their muscles resulting in a severe loss of energy and muscle that burns fat. If, in your weight management plan, you are tempted to count calories, count proteins instead and make sure you get enough.

While meat is a great source of protein and is a complete protein, not all meat is good for you. Imagine a big ole chicken fried steak made from processed hamburger meat, fried in deep fat. It stands no comparison to a grass-fed, organic steak that is free from chemicals, hormones and fat. Paying attention to what happens between the source of your protein and when you actually put it on your plate is helpful in determining if it is, in fact, really beneficial for you.

Fats

Fats have a bad rap when it comes to dieting. Even the word oozes with calories and just sounds like dimples on your thighs. But fats are a necessary part of a healthy diet. Not only do fats work to keep your body warm, they also provide energy, support healthy cell growth and assist in absorbing nutrients into your system. If you want to find out what fats do for hormones, block them out of your diet. You will be a raving maniac. Fats are, in no uncertain terms, ultra important in your diet.

There are different kinds of fats, though. That is where the confusion comes in. There are good fats, bad fats, trans fats, saturated fats, monounsaturated fats and polyunsaturated fats. Now, you're really confused!

Basically it boils down to this, there are four kinds of fats. Saturated fats and Trans fats are the bad guys. They solidify when stored at room temperature like a stick of butter does. Monounsaturated and polyunsaturated fats are found in vegetable oils and those that are generally more liquid-like.

Bad fats raise your cholesterol levels. They can be a culprit behind heart conditions, high blood pressure and obesity. Good fats can help to lower the levels. Even good fats should be eaten wisely though and in moderation.

Polyunsaturated fats fall into one of two groups. There is the Omega-3 category and those with Omega-6. While both are needed in a balanced diet and neither can be produced strictly within the body, it is a proven fact that Americans consume way too much Omega-6's which is evident in many health conditions such as heart problems, cancer and asthma. Examples of Omega-6 are corn oil and cottonseed oil. Omega-3 is found in nuts and fish. It is has also been proven that an imbalance of Omega-3 and Omega-6 can lead to disorders such as depression, dyslexia and obesity.

Coconut oil is becoming a popular fat to use. It can actually help the body get rid of fat and is quite healthy too. It promotes good heart health, boosts the immune system, supports healthy skin and teeth, is a fantastic anti-aging remedy, promotes energy and is a solution to thyroid issues as well. Coconut oil fries well and can often be substituted in baking without much notice. Look for brands that are unprocessed and cold pressed and of course, organic.

FRUITS AND FIBER (AND VEGGIES TOO)

Fiber is another must in a healthy diet. It helps the body rid itself of wastes, is essential in prevention of certain diseases and is a great tool for weight loss. Fiber makes us feel full and satisfied. Insoluble fiber can be found in nuts, whole grains, wheat bran, and in many vegetables. Soluble fiber can even be found in fruits, beans and barley grains. Eating foods that contain fiber is a great weight management strategy.

H20

It's so simple, it almost seems unreal. Water is a dieter's best friend. It energizes, rids the body of waste and fat, helps the body actually burn fat and can boost your metabolism. Furthermore, it helps make us feel full. What's not to love about water?

Generally when you don't want water or don't like the taste, it's because you are not drinking enough of it. One sign of dehydration is feeling like you do not want water. Of course, that makes matters worse.

The body is made up of water, about 60% to be exact. Water makes up 85% of our brain. It is life or death. You have to have water to survive. It is estimated that as many as 75% of the American population is dehydrated. When we are thirsty, we grab a soda.

It is recommended that the average person drink about eight glasses of water a day. If you are very large, exercising a lot or are in extreme weather conditions, you will need more. It is best to count your intake rather than to rely on thirst alone so that you are sure to get enough.

Water is another thing that is not created equally. Tap water is known to be loaded with contaminates and chemicals so if you are going to drink out of the tap, purchase a good quality water filter. Bottled water can vary too so do your homework on which brands to trust.

You can follow your gut too. Some water brands do not set well for some which is a good indication to avoid those.

Water is on your side. It will help you reach your weight management goals. Dive in!

So...I Can Eat Whatever I Want?

In figuring proportions for specific body types, it just makes sense to measure them out with your own body. Generally, one serving is a handful but since our hands are different sizes, you may find it helpful to use your own hand to determine what a portion is for your size and build. Also, please note some examples of food sources. Healthy high protein foods include: lean beef, turkey, lamb, chicken, beans, nut butter, fish, cashews, pecans, peanuts, sunflower seeds and pumpkin seeds. High carbohydrates foods can be best attained through eating less-processed, closer-to-nature sources such as sweet potatoes, bagels, whole grain bread, raisins and pasta. Likewise, chose fat dense foods that are beneficial and not harmful like avocados, coconut oil, nuts and olives. Needless to say, vegetables are best when organic and are as fresh as possible, preferably locally grown. The less vegetables are cooked, the better.

For our purposes, men and women have different recommendations. The male and female bodies metabolize differently and are since males are often times larger, we have customized the chart accordingly.

Another note is that all body types can and should have carbs, proteins, fats and protein. The secret to success is found in the ratios. Your body will follow the lead once you get the rhythm down. Soon you will begin to see that the things want are the things you should be having and that when you have had enough, you will be full. We cannot expect our bodies to react that way when we are not giving them the right foods in the right proportions. You are going to love the difference eating according to your body type will make.

Let's do a quick reminder on body types. Then go over the quantity of carbs, protein and fats to optimize each body type.

The Body Type Breakdown

Ectomorphs

Bodily Characteristics

- Smaller bone structure
- Thin limbs
- Small shoulders, chest and buttocks
- Difficulty building muscle
- High metabolism
- High Carbohydrate Tolerance

Ecotmorph Diet

Carbs, carbs, carbs. An Ectomorph thrives on carbohydrates and utilizes them well. They rarely note a sugar spike or have difficulty with insulin because they actually use the energy. They do best with a medium protein and low fat diet. Portions of approximately 55% carbohydrates, 25% protein, and 20% fat has been proven to be very effective with this body type.

An example of a meal plan for an Ectomorph man:

- 2 palms of food packed with protein
- 2 fists of vegetables
- 2 cupped handfuls of carbohydrates rich food
- 1 thumb of high fat food
-

An Ectomorph woman should do well with:

- 1 palm of food packed with protein
- 1 fists of vegetables
- 2 cupped handfuls of carbohydrates rich food
- 1/2 thumb of high fat food

Ectomorphs are high energy people so for exercise, running, jogging and bicycling are all super activities.

Mesomorphs

- Medium bone structure
- Muscle bound limbs
- Broad shoulders
- High muscle throughout body
- Build muscle easily
- Burn fat easily

The best diet ratio for a Mesomorph seems to be 40% carbs, 30% of both fat and protein.

Here's a great eating plan for a Mesomorph man:

- 2 palms of food packed with protein
- 2 fists of vegetables
- 2 cupped handfuls of carbohydrates rich food
- 2 thumbs of high fat food

An excellent meal for a Mesomorph woman would be:
- 1 palm of food packed with protein
- 1 fists of vegetables
- 1 cupped handfuls of carbohydrates rich food
- 1 thumb of high fat food

Muscle sculpting and muscle building are great exercises for Mesomorphs as well as circuit training.

Endomorphs
- **Large Bone Structure**
- **Tendency to Retain Fat**
- **Difficulty in Losing Weight**
- **Gain Weight Easily**

They do not do well with excess calories nor do they burn carbs well so if this is your body type, all or in part, be encouraged. Knowing more about it will help you by leaps and bounds.

With a diet of 40% fat, 35% protein and 25% carbohydrates, you should be well on your way to that fabulous you.

A well balance meal plan for an Endomorph man includes:

- 2 palms of foods rich in protein
- 2 fists of vegetables
- 1 cupped handful of carbohydrates
- 3 thumbs of foods high in fat

A healthy meal plan for an Endomorph female would be:

- 1 palm of protein rich foods
- 1 fist of vegetables
- 1/2 cupped handful of foods high in carbohydrates
- 2 thumbs of foods high in fat

Great exercises for Endomorphs include moderate aerobics like walking fast, light jogging, swimming and stationary bicycling.

CRANKING UP YOUR METABOLISM (FOR ANY BODY TYPE)

No, no, don't put the book down yet. The best has been saved for last. Exercise, also known as the "E" word, is really our friend. It is what sets the plan in motion. It's like the icing on the cake. It will put the exclamation mark on your weight management eating plan. It will not only make you look better, you will feel better too. But until the energizing comes, you will have to ride on faith.

The most important thing when choosing an exercise program is to find one that works for you. What do you like to do? What do you hate to do? How much time do you have? How much are you willing, or do you need, to put into it?

If you hate to run but love to dance, an aerobics class may be for you. But if you have two left feet, you may opt for water exercises instead. There are a myriad of exercises and you are sure to find one that will fit your liking as well as your personality and your schedule as well.

Group Exercise vs. Individual Plans

Let's face it. Some of us are introverts and some of us are extroverts. There are those of us who would not be happy to walk the block alone, much less a mile or two. Then there are the quieter types who do their deepest thinking when left to sweat alone. Maybe you are in-between and function best with a buddy. Whatever it is that makes you tick, seek your exercise option accordingly.

The Gym

Going to the gym has its benefits for sure. Usually there is a fee which for some can be a drawback but for others offers just the commitment needed to get in gear. Generally at a gym, a staff member will show you the ropes the first time or two and it's up to you to put your program together accordingly. Again, that works wonderfully for some, but others may need to enlist with a personal trainer. Usually there are optional group sessions that take place too.

Aerobics

Aerobics are great for the heart and for weight loss and getting in shape. If you are one that likes to kick it with dancing and music, you will have so much fun, you won't even realize you are exercising. It's a great way to burn calories and turn flab into muscle. And if you don't like to strut your stuff in the company of others, grab a DVD and do aerobics in the privacy of your own home.

Water Exercise Class

For those that have medical limitations or just love the water, exercises can be done in the pool. Water makes for low impact but the results are usually astounding. YMCAs often offer water work-outs at low cost and generally have beginner, intermediate and advanced levels.

The Peak Plan

The Peak Fitness Plan is a fairly new concept that is taking the nation by a storm. It is a scientifically proven way to exercise that requires little time but it big on results.
There are variations of this plan but the jest of it is to warm up for 3 minutes then, to exercise with all of your might for 30 seconds. During this time you will want to reach your peak heart rate. For 90 seconds you will cool down by moving at a slower pace. Then, once again, work as hard as you can for 30 seconds and cool down. Then again. The goal is to do the cycle 8 times, 3 times a week, reaching your anaerobic threshold during the peaks. That is determined by subtracting your age from 220. You can purchase a heart rate monitor that will calculate your heart rate.
Most people will not be able to go the full round of the work-out but can steadily build up to it. For the workout, you can chose whatever activity that you prefer that gets your heart pumping. A stationary bike, treadmill, even running in place are all good options.

Doing Your Own Thing

Some of us just don't conform to any given class or program. We want to do it our own way. That is fine and you may see even better results this way but you are going to have to be very self-disciplined. The key will be to find something that you love to do, that really gives your body a great workout and that you have access to do at least three times a week.

Swimming, snow skiing, jogging and tennis are all fun things that can be done on your own. You will want to set productive and attainable goals and lay down some rules for yourself but if you are that person…go for it!

IT'S TIME TO DO THIS ONCE AND FOR ALL!

Losing weight is a life style, it's about choices and making the ones that are right for you. An effective diet has little or nothing to do with counting calories, stepping onto the scale or torturing yourself. It for sure has nothing to do with starving.

Shedding unwanted pounds and getting into shape boils down to an attitude of the heart and loving yourself thin. Spend time with yourself and discover what makes you tick and what ticks you off. Know your triggers, your weaknesses and your strengths.

Most importantly, get to know your body type. Working within the realistic realms of your personal body type or types will help prevent dangerous pitfalls and deep depression that often goes hand-in-hand with dieting. Managing your weight by realizing and embracing your body style is empowering. It is invigorating and encouraging.

Miraculously, when you know yourself inside and out, physically, emotionally and even spiritually, you will be able to take charge of your life and reinvent yourself accordingly. Want to drop a few pounds? Do it! Want to get in tip-top shape? Do it! The power is all yours when you take your fate into your own hands with the simple steps you have now discovered.

All the best,
Elaina Moore

P.S. Don't forget, I want to reach as many people as possible with this message of "How to Stop Yo-Yo Dieting so please don't forget to leave this book a 5 start review on Amazon!

www.ingramcontent.com/pod-product-compliance
Lightning Source LLC
Chambersburg PA
CBHW070509290526
45790CB00003B/1168